Keto Diet Cookbook 2019-2020

Easy & Most Delicious Recipes to Lose Weight, Balance Hormones, Boost Brain Health, and Reverse Disease

By
Melissa Tristan

Copyright © **Melissa Tristan** 2019

All rights reserved. No part of this publication maybe reproduced, stored or transmitted in any form or by any means, electronic, mechanical, photocopying, recording, scanning, or otherwise without written permission from the author. It is illegal to copy this book, post it to a website, or distribute it by any other means without permission.

Melissa Tristan moral right to be identified as the author of this work.

Table of Contents

★★ Keto Bread Recipes 5

Fat Head Pizza Crust 5

Cauliflower Pizza Crust 6

1-Minute Keto Muffins 9

Low Carb Naan 10

Low Carb Chocolate Muffins 11

Cheesy Garlic Bread Muffins 13

Keto-Friendly Fathead Cinnamon Rolls 15

Keto Pretzels Recipe - Homemade Soft Pretzel - Low Carb & Gluten Free 16

Keto Blueberry Lemon Bread 19

Keto Fathead Rolls 22

Keto Bread 23

Low Carb Tortillas 24

The Best Cloud Bread Recipe 26

Keto Focaccia Bread Recipe 27

Nearly No Carb Keto Bread 30

Savory Italian Crackers 31

Keto Garlic Chia Crackers Recipe 32

Keto Italian Flaxseed Crackers Recipe 34

Keto Pull Apart Pizza Bread Recipe 35

Keto Flatbread Recipe..39

Zucchini Coconut Bread..41

Indian Fry Bread (Low Carb)...42

Low Carb and Keto Fluffy Waffles Recipe 45

Low Carb Keto Bagels Recipe (Fathead Dough) 47

★★ Keto Bread Recipes

Fat Head Pizza Crust

Prep+Cook Time: 30 mins, Servings: 8

Ingredients

- 1 1/2 cups shredded mozzarella
- 3/4 cup almond flour
- 2 tablespoons of cream cheese, cubed
- 1 egg
- garlic powder, onion powder, and mixed herbs for seasoning

Instructions

- Put Mozzarella and cream cheese in a medium bowl
- Microwave for 1 min, stir and then another 30 sec, stir
- Stir in egg and almond flour
- Wet hands and spread "dough" thin on parchment paper. It should spread evenly with dough-like consistency.
- Poke rows of holes with a fork to avoid bubbles.
- Put in 425-degree oven
- After 8 minutes check the crust and poke holes if there are bubbles.

- Add desired pizza toppings.
- Continue cooking for a total of 12 to 14 minutes or until slightly brown and golden.

Nutrition Info : Serving Size: 1 slice , Calories: 143 , Sugar: 1g , Sodium: 346mg , Fat: 12g , Carbohydrates: 2g , Fiber: 1g , Protein: 9g

Cauliflower Pizza Crust

Prep+Cook Time: 35 minutes, Servings: 8 slices

Ingredients

- 1 small to medium sized head of cauliflower - should make 2 cups once processed ((many stores now sell frozen riced cauliflower)
- 1/2 teaspoon dried basil
- 1/4 teaspoon dried oregano
- 1 teaspoon garlic salt OR 1/4 teaspoon salt and 1/4 teaspoon garlic powder ((I love Lawry's))
- 1/3 cup shredded parmesan cheese
- 1/3 cup mozzarella cheese
- 1 egg
- pizza sauce & toppings of your choice

Instructions

- Preheat oven to 450 degrees
- Place a piece of parchment paper on a cookie sheet and spray it with non-stick butter spray. (or use a silicon baking mat, which is my favorite thing in the world)
- Cut off the florets of the cauliflower - try to cut off as much of the stem as possible. Place the florets in a food processor and "rice it" - you do this by pulsing the food processor - press the button in short "pulse-like" increments- be very careful not to over process and puree, it won't be good!
- The cauliflower should come out looking almost grain like. See picture.
- (You can save a step by buying the frozen riced cauliflower. I have done this and it comes out just as good!)
- Place the cauliflower in a microwave safe bowl and microwave it for about 4 minutes.
- Pour it out on a kitchen towel or paper towels and wring the water out of it. The more water you get out the better.
- Place in a bowl and mix in all of the other ingredients.
- Using your hands, take the mixture and make it into a ball.

- Place it on the parchment paper and flatten it out to a pizza shape. (careful not too make it too thick or thin!)
- Place the cookie sheet in the oven and bake until the edges start to get golden brown and the middle sets - about 15 minutes. Flip over and bake another few minutes.
- Remove from oven and let it cool for a few minutes.
- Put your favorite pizza sauce and toppings on and cook on 350 degrees for 3-5 minutes or until cheese is melting and starting to brown.
- If you have a pizza stone, I think this would help it to get nice and crispy, I don't have one, but I may have to invest in one!

Nutrition Info: Calories: 53kcal , Fat: 2g , Saturated fat: 1g , Cholesterol: 26mg , Carbohydrates: 1g , Protein: 3g

1-Minute Keto Muffins

Prep+Cook Time: 2 mins, Servings:4

Ingredients

- 1 egg
- 2 tsp coconut flour or more depending on brand used
- pinch baking soda , pinch salt

Instructions

- Grease a ramekin dish (or very large coffee mug) with coconut oil or butter.
- Mix all the ingredients together with a fork to ensure it is lump free.
- Cook the 1-minute keto muffin in the microwave on HIGH for 45 seconds - 1 minute. Alternatively, they can be baked in an oven, at 200C/400F for 12 minutes.
- Cut in half and serve. (toasting or frying is optional)

Nutrition Info : Calories 113 Calories from Fat 54 , Total Fat 6g 9% , Saturated Fat 2g 10% , Cholesterol 186mg 62% , Total Carbohydrates 5g 2% , Dietary Fiber 3g 12% , Protein 7g

Low Carb Naan

Prep+Cook Time: 35 minutes, Servings: 2 servings

Ingredients

- 1/2 cup Coconut flour
- 1.5 tbsp psyllium husk powder
- 2 tbsp coconut oil
- 1/4 tsp baking powder
- 1-1.5 cups hot water
- 1 Tbsp minced garlic (optional)
- 1/4 tsp Pink Himalayan Salt

Instructions

- Combine the coconut flour, psyillium husk powder, baking powder, salt and coconut oil. Add the minced garlic to the mixture.
- Add 1 cup of hot water to start and combine. Add more hot water if needed. If the consistency is too wet add more psyllium husk powder
- Knead with your hands for a minute and let it sit in a bowl for 15 minutes.

- Pull apart the dough into as big or as little balls as you like and roll out using some parchment paper a rolling pin.
- Heat a skillet to medium heat and add a naan to the heated skillet. Flip after a couple minutes (it will be brown on the other side), and cook until browned on both sides.
- Tip: If the naan starts to puff up, you know its done!
- Complete until all naans are cooked and enjoy!

Nutrition Info: Calories: 271kcal, Carbohydrates: 25g, Protein: 4g, Fat: 17.5g, Fiber: 19g

Low Carb Chocolate Muffins

Prep+Cook Time: 30 minutes, Servings: 12 muffins

Ingredients

- 1/2 cup peanut flour
- 1/4 cup Unsweetened Cocoa Powder
- 1 ounce Unsweetened Bakers Chocolate
- 1 ounce Lily's Chocolate Chips
- 1/4 cup erythritol
- 1/4 cup Heavy Cream

- 4 large eggs
- 1 tsp Baking powder
- 4 tbsp Butter
- 1 tsp vanilla extract
- 1/8 tsp Pink Himalayan Salt

Instructions

- Start by combining dry ingredients. Thoroughly mix peanut flour, cocoa powder, erythritol, baking powder and salt.
- In a separate bowl combine heavy cream and butter with a hand mixer.
- Once combined add eggs and vanilla and mix until combined.
- Add the dry ingredients to the wet and mix until combined.
- Add all of the bakers chocolate and HALF of the Lilly's chocolate and fold together.
- Scoop into muffin tins and top with the remaining Lilly's chocolate.
- Bake at 350 for 20 minutes. Test with a toothpick. Enjoy!

Nutrition Info: Calories: 112kcal, Carbohydrates: 4g, Protein: 6g, Fat: 9g, Fiber: 2g

Cheesy Garlic Bread Muffins

Prep+Cook Time 45 mins, Servings: 12

Ingredients

- 6 tbsp butter melted
- 5 cloves garlic pressed or finely minced, divided
- 1/2 cup sour cream
- 4 large eggs
- 1 tsp salt
- 3 cups almond flour
- 2 tsp baking powder
- 1 cup shredded Cheddar cheese I used Cabot Seriously Sharp
- 1/4 cup chopped parsley
- 4 ounces shredded mozzarella
- Sea salt for sprinkling

Instructions

- Preheat the oven to 325F and grease a standard-size non-stick muffin tin very well. Set the muffin tin on a large rimmed baking sheet (to catch the drips).
- Combine the melted butter and 3 cloves of the garlic. Set aside.
- In a high-powered blender or a food processor, combine the sour cream, eggs, remaining garlic, and salt. Process until well combined. Add the almond flour, baking powder, cheese, and parsley and process again until smooth.
- Divide half of the batter between the prepared muffin cups and use a spoon to make a small well in the center of each.
- Divide the shredded mozzarella between the muffins, pressing into the wells. Drizzle with about 1 tsp of the garlic butter mixture.
- Divide the remaining batter between each muffin cup, make sure to cover the cheese as best you can. Brush the tops with the remaining garlic butter and sprinkle with sea salt.
- Bake 25 minutes or so, until tops are golden brown and just firm to the touch. These will drip a lot of oil as they

bake and it may spill over the sides a bit (hence the baking sheet underneath - to save your oven!).
- o Remove and let cool 10 minutes before serving. They are fantastic still warm from the oven with the cheese still gooey. They are great cool too and warm up nicely.

Nutrition Info : Calories 322 Calories from Fat 245 , Total Fat 27.17g 42% , Saturated Fat 9.34g 47% , Total Carbohydrates 7.44g 2% , Dietary Fiber 3.07g 12% , Protein 12.83g

Keto-Friendly Fathead Cinnamon Rolls

Prep+Cook Time: 20 mins, Servings: 10

Ingredients: -Roll:

- 6 oz Mozzarella Cheese
- 3 oz Almond flour
- 2 tbsp cream cheese , 1 egg
- 1/4 tsp baking powder
- 3 Tbsp Monkfruit Erythritol blend , 1 Tbsp Cinnamon
- I revised this based on feedback below
- 3 Tbsp melted butter or Ghee

Cream Cheese Frosting:

- 2 oz Cream cheese , 1 tsp Cinnamon , 1 Tbsp Monkfruit Erythritol blend

Instructions
- o Preheat oven to 400 F
- o In a microwave safe bowl add mozzarella, almond flour, and baking powder and toss to combine.
- o Next, add cream cheese and microwave for 60 seconds, take out and mix, microwave for another 30 seconds, and then mix again. Then, add egg and mix until dough forms. Take the dough and place in between 2 sheets of parchment paper, and roll out to 1/4 inch thickness.
- o Spread melted butter over the dough, then evenly sprinkle cinnamon and erythritol.
- o Roll into jellyroll shape, making sure to keep it as tight as possible, then slice off half in rounds, and place on a baking sheet lined with parchment paper or a sil pat and place about 1 inch apart.
- o Bake at 400F until rolls are puffed and brown 10-15 mins, however, keep an eye on them as they can burn quickly.
- o While rolls are baking mix frosting ingredients together.

Nutrition Info : Calories 194kcal

Keto Pretzels Recipe - Homemade Soft Pretzel - Low Carb & Gluten Free

Prep+Cook Time: 32 minutes, Servings: 12

Ingredients

- 3 cups mozzarella cheese shredded
- 4 tablespoons Cream Cheese
- 1 1/2 cups almond flour
- 2 teaspoons xanthum gum
- 2 eggs room temperature
- 2 teaspoons dried yeast approxiamtely 1 sachet
- 2 tablespoons warm water
- 2 tablespoon Butter melted
- 1 tablespoon pretzel salt

Instructions

- Preheat oven to 200C/390F.
- In a microwave safe dish, place the mozzarella cheese and cream cheese and microwave in 30 sec increments, stirring in between, until fully melted and almost liquid.
- Dissolve the yeast in the warm water and allow it to sit and activate for 2 minutes.
- In your stand mixer (using the dough hook attachment), place the almond meal and xanthum gum and mix well.

- Add the eggs, yeast mixture and 1 tablespoon of the melted butter and mix well.
- Add the hot melted cheese to the stand mixer and allow it to knead the dough until all the ingredients are fully combined. Around 5-10 minutes.
- Split the dough into 12 balls. The dough is easiest to work with while it is warm.
- Roll each ball into a long skinny log and twist into a pretzel shape. Place on a lined cookie sheet and give a little space with side as the pretzels will rise.
- Brush the pretzels with the remaining butter and sprinkle with pretzel salt.
- Bake in the oven for 12-15 minutes.
- When the pretzels are golden brown, remove them from the oven, and don't burn your fingers trying to eat them immediately.

Nutrition Info: Calories: 217kcal, Carbohydrates: 3g, Protein: 11g, Fat: 18g, Saturated Fat: 7g, Polyunsaturated Fat: 2g

Keto Blueberry Lemon Bread

Prep+Cook Time: 1 hour 25 minutes, Servings: 12

Ingredients

Keto Blueberry Lemon Bread Batter

- 2 1/2 cups of finely milled almond flour
- 1 cup of sugar substitute
- 2 teaspoons of baking powder
- 1/2 teaspoon of sea salt
- 8 whole eggs
- 8 ounces of room temperature full-fat cream cheese
- 2 teaspoons of lemon extract
- 1/2 cup of room temperature unsalted butter
- 2 cups of fresh or frozen whole blueberries
- 1 tablespoon of lemon zest

Keto Lemon Glaze

- 3/4 cup of confectioners sugar substitute
- 3 tablespoons of freshly squeezed lemon juice
- 2 tablespoons of heavy whipping cream

- 1 teaspoon of lemon extract
- 2 teaspoons of lemon zest

Instructions -Keto Blueberry Lemon Bread

- Preheat oven to 350 degrees.
- Grease and line with parchment paper a 10X5 inch loaf pan or two 6 inch loaf pans. (note if using two smaller pans check for doneness at 35 minute mark)
- In a medium-sized bowl measure then sift the almond flour. To the sifted flour add the baking powder, sea salt and stir. Set this aside.
- In a large bowl using an electric hand-held mixer or stand-up mixer blend the butter, cream cheese, and sugar-substitute until mixture is light fluffy.
- Next add the 8 eggs one at a time, making sure to scrape the bowl several times.
- To the wet batter add the dry ingredients and combine until well-incorporated.
- Fold in the blueberries into the bread batter.
- Spread the batter into the greased loaf pan.
- Bake for 60-70 minutes or until an inserted toothpick comes out clean.
- Allow the loaf to cool in the pan for about 30 minutes before taking it out of the pan. Then let the pan cool on a baking rack

for at least 60 minutes before adding the icing, refrigerating or freezing.

Keto Lemon Glaze

- To make the lemon glaze imply combine the confectioners sugar substitute, lemon juice, lemon extract, lemon zest and heavy whipping cream. Stir until fully incorporated.

Nutrition Info : Calories: 350 Total Fat: 30.6g Saturated Fat: 11.4g, Protein: 10.3g

Keto Fathead Rolls

Prep+Cook Time 25 minutes, Servings 4 People

Ingredients

- 2 oz cream cheese , 3/4 cup shredded mozzarella
- 1 egg beaten , 1/4 tsp garlic powder
- 1/3 cup almond flour , 2 tsp baking powder
- 1/2 cup shredded cheddar cheese

Instructions

- Preheat the oven to 425°
- In a small bowl, add cream cheese and mozzarella. Microwave on high for 20 seconds at a time until melted.
- In a separate bowl, whisk egg until beaten. Add dry ingredients and mix well.
- Work mozzarella/cc mixture into dough. Dough will be sticky. Stir in cheddar cheese.
- Spoon dough onto plastic wrap. Dust the top of it with almond flour.
- Fold the plastic wrap over the dough and gently start working into a ball.
- Cover and refrigerate 30 minutes.

- Cut dough ball into 4. Roll each section into a ball the ball in half. This is your top and bottom bun
- Sit cut side down on parchment paper or very well greased sheet pan.
- Bake 10-12 minutes or until golden and set up.

Nutrition Info : Calories 160

Keto Bread

Prep+Cook Time 55 Mins

Ingredients

- 100 g Butter melted (3.5 oz / 1/2 cup)
- 30 g Coconut Oil (1 oz / 2 Tbsp)
- 7 Large Eggs (50g / 1.7 oz each)
- 1 teaspoon baking powder (5g / 0.2 oz)
- 200 g Almond Flour (7 oz / 2 Cups)
- 1/2 teaspoon xanthan gum (2g)
- 1/2 teaspoon Salt (2g)

Instructions

- Preheat oven to 180 c (355 F)

- o Put the eggs into a bowl and beat for 1 - 2 mins on high.
- o Add coconut oil and melted butter to eggs, continue beating.
- o Add remaining ingredients. Will become quite thick
- o Scrape into a loaf pan lined with baking paper.
- o Bake for 45 minutes. (Remove once a skewer comes out of the middle clean).
- o Slice into 16 thin slices, and store in an airtight container in the fridge for up to 7 days, or up to 1 month in the freezer.

Nutrition Info : Calories 165 Calories from Fat 135 , Total Fat 15g 23% , Saturated Fat 4.8g 24% , Total Carbohydrates 3g 1% , Dietary Fiber 1.5g 6% , Protein 6g 12%

Low Carb Tortillas

Prep+Cook Time: 20 minutes, Servings: 16 Tortillas

Ingredients

- 8 large Egg Whites , 1/3 cup Coconut flour
- 10 tbsp Water , 1/4 tsp Baking powder
- 1/4 tsp garlic powder , 1/4 tsp Onion powder
- 1/4 tsp chili powder

- 1/4 tsp Pink Himalayan Salt

Instructions
- Add egg whites, coconut flour, baking powder and water in a bowl. Combine well (should be a uniform, watery mixture).
- Optional: add seasonings and mix.
- Heat a skillet (any size you want your tortillas to be) to low heat. Wait until the pan is hot, spray with cooking spray, and drop some of the mixture into the center (i like to use a 1/4 measuring cup).
- As quickly as possible tilt the skillet on all edge to spread the batter as thin as possible. You can always add more in the areas not covered.
- Allow it to cook for a couple minutes until it starts to rise/bubble or you lift it up and the other side has browned. Flip and cook for 1 additional minute.
- Repeat process until all the batter is cooked. The above mixture made 16 small taco sized tortillas for us.
- TIP: If your first tortilla doesn't spread thin enough on the skillet (comes out more like a pancake) add more water to the egg white mixture and mix!

Nutrition Info: Calories: 75kcal, Carbohydrates: 6g, Protein: 8.5g, Fat: 1.5g, Fiber: 3.25g

The Best Cloud Bread Recipe

Prep+Cook Time 25 mins

Ingredients

- 4 large eggs, separated
- 1/2 teaspoon cream of tartar
- 2 ounces low-fat cream cheese
- 1 teaspoon Italian herb seasoning
- 1/2 teaspoon sea salt
- 1/4 - 1/2 teaspoon garlic powder

Instructions

- Preheat the oven to 300 degrees F. If you have a convection oven, set on convect. Line two large baking sheets with parchment paper.
- Separate the egg whites and egg yolks. Place the whites in a stand mixer with a whip attachment. Add the cream of tartar and beat on high until the froth turns into firm meringue peaks. Move to a separate bowl.
- Place the cream cheese in the empty stand mixing bowl. Beat on high to soften. Then add the egg yolks one at a

time to incorporate. Scrape the bowl and beat until the mixture is completely smooth. Then beat in the Italian seasoning, salt, and garlic powder.
- Gently fold the firm meringue into the yolk mixture. Try to deflate the meringue as little as possible, so the mixture is still firm and foamy. Spoon 1/4 cup portions of the foam onto the baking sheets and spread into even 4-inch circles, 3/4 inch high. Make sure to leave space around each circle.
- Bake on convect for 15-18 minutes, or in a conventional oven for up to 30 minutes. The bread should be golden on the outside and firm. The center should not jiggle when shaken. Cool for several minutes on the baking sheets, then move and serve!

Nutrition Info : Calories 36 Calories from Fat 18 , Total Fat 2g 3% , Saturated Fat 1g 5% , Cholesterol 68mg 23% , Sugars 0g , Protein 2g 4%

Keto Focaccia Bread Recipe

Prep+Time: 25 minutes, Servings: 1

Ingredients

- 2 Tablespoons (12 g) gelatin powder
- 2 Tablespoons (30 ml) water
- 2 Tablespoons (30 ml) hot water
- 1 Tablespoon (8 g) Nutrition Infoal yeast flakes
- 1 cup (240 ml) hot water
- 2 cups (8 oz or 225 g) coconut flour
- 1/4 cup (0.9 oz or 25 g) psyllium husk powder
- 1 teaspoon (2 g) baking powder
- 1 teaspoon (4 g) baking soda
- Dash of garlic powder
- Dash of salt
- 3 large eggs
- 2 teaspoons (10 ml) olive oil
- Handful of fresh rosemary tips
- Sea salt flakes

Instructions

Preheat the oven to 350 F (175 C).
- Make a gelatine egg by sprinkling the gelatine powder over two tablespoons water. Once dissolved, stir in two tablespoons boiling hot water and set aside while you prepare the remaining ingredients.
- Dissolve the Nutrition Infoal yeast flakes in a cup of hot water and set aside.

- o Combine the coconut flour, psyllium husk powder, baking powder, baking soda, garlic powder and salt in a bowl.
- o In a separate bowl, whisk the eggs with the olive oil and add in the gelatine mixture once it has cooled slightly (else it will scramble the eggs). Check the temperature of the nutritional yeast water, once that has sufficiently cooled to add to the egg mixture, whisk this in too.
- o Add the egg mixture to the flour mixture and combine well. Tip the mixture into a greased baking dish (approx. 6-in x 6-in) so the mixture comes up at least an inch high. Make small indentations using the back of a chopstick and pierce with little washed rosemary tips.
- o Bake in the oven for 25 minutes, or until a cake tester inserted comes out clean. Scatter over sea salt flakes and trim into pieces once cooled.

Nutrition Info: Calories: 212 Sugar: 3 g Fat: 9 g Carbohydrates: 17 g Fiber: 14 g Protein: 13 g

Nearly No Carb Keto Bread

Prep+Cook Time 31 minutes, Servings 12

Ingredients

- 8 ounces cream cheese
- 2 cups mozzarella cheese grated (about 210 grams)
- 3 large eggs
- 1/4 cup parmesan cheese grated (about 27 grams)
- 1 cup crushed pork rinds about 46 grams
- 1 tablespoon baking powder

Optional: - herbs and spices to taste

Instructions

- Preheat oven to 375°F. Line baking sheet (I used a 12 x 17 jelly roll pan) with parchment paper.
- Place cream cheese and mozzarella cheese in large microwaveable bowl.
- Microwave cheese on high power for one minute, stir, then microwave for another minute and stir again. The cheese should be fully melted.

- o Add egg, parmesan, pork rinds, and baking powder. Stir until all ingredients have been incorporated.
- o Spread mixture onto parchment paper lined pan. Bake at 375°F for 15-20 or until lightly brown on top.
- o Allow pan to cool on rack for 15 minutes, then remove bread from pan and cool directly on rack.
- o Slice into 12 equal sized pieces. Can be eaten plain or used to make sandwiches.

Nutrition Info : Calories 166 Calories from Fat 117, Total Fat 13g 20% , Saturated Fat 7g 35% , Cholesterol 86mg 29% , Sodium 294mg 12% , Potassium 158mg 5%, Total Carbohydrates 1g 0% , Dietary Fiber 0g 0% ,Sugars 0g

Savory Italian Crackers

PrepCook Time 25 minutes, Servings: 4

Ingredients

- 1-1/2 cups (143 g) Almond Flour
- 1 Egg
- 2 Tbsp (30 ml) Olive Oil
- 3/4 tsp (5 g) Salt

- 1/4 tsp (0.5 g) Basil
- 1/2 tsp (1 g) Thyme
- 1/4 tsp (0.5 g) Oregano
- 1/2 tsp (1 g) Onion Powder
- 1/4 tsp (0.5 g) Garlic Powder

Instructions

- Preheat oven to 350°F (177°C).
- Mix all the ingredients well to form a dough.
- Shape dough into a long rectangular log (use some foil or cling film to pack the dough tight) and then cut into thin slices (approximately 0.2 inches (0.5 cm) thick). Gently place each slice onto a parchment paper lined baking tray. It makes approx. 20-30 crackers, depending on size.
- Bake for 10-12 minutes.

Nutrition Info : Calories: 1011kcal, Carbohydrates: 29g, Protein: 31g

Keto Garlic Chia Crackers Recipe

Prep+Cook Time: 30 minutes, Servings: 4

Ingredients

- 1/2 cup (60 g) chia or flax meal (use chia or flax seed, and use a coffee grinder or a good blender to process into a flour first)
- 1 egg, whisked , 2 Tablespoons chia seeds (24 g)
- 1 Tablespoon garlic powder (10 g) , 1 teaspoon salt (5 g)

Instructions

- Preheat oven to 300F (150 C).
- In a mixing bowl, combine all the ingredients.
- Place a piece of parchment paper on a flat surface. Place the dough on top of the paper and place another piece of parchment paper on top of the dough.
- Use a rolling pin to roll the dough to desired thickness (approx. 0.2 cm thick).
- Carefully pull the top piece of parchment paper away and use a sharp knife to score the dough into small cracker squares.
- Place the parchment paper with the scored dough on a baking tray and bake for 30 minutes.

- o Break the crackers apart after 15 minutes and flip the crackers over.

Nutrition Info : Calories: 123 Sugar: 1 g Fat: 9 g Carbohydrates: 8 g Fiber: 5 g Protein: 6 g

Keto Italian Flaxseed Crackers Recipe

PrepCook Time: 20 minutes, Servings: 4

Ingredients

- 1 cup (112 g) flaxseeds, ground into a meal (use a food processor, blender, or coffee grinder)
- ½ cup (120 ml) water
- 1 Tablespoon (10 g) garlic powder
- 2 teaspoons (5 g) onion powder
- 1 Tablespoon (3 g) Italian seasoning
- 1 teaspoon (5 g) salt

Instructions

- o Heat oven to 400 F (200 C).

U In a medium mixing bowl, combine flaxseed with spices. Add water and stir until combined. Knead for a few minutes.
- Place the dough onto a large piece of parchment paper on a flat surface. Place another piece of parchment paper on top of the dough.
- Use a rolling pin to roll the dough to desired thickness (approx. 0.3 cm).
- Gently pull the top piece of parchment paper away from the dough. Use a sharp knife, or pizza cutter and score the flattened dough into cracker size pieces.
- Place the parchment paper with the scored dough onto a baking tray and bake for 10-15 minutes (they should be easy to lift off the parchment paper but not crunchy).
- Carefully pull the crackers apart and flip them over.
- Reduce oven heat to 300 F (150 C).
- Bake for another 15-20 minutes until crispy but not burnt.

Nutrition Info : Calories: 151, Sugar: 1 g Fat: 12 g, Carbohydrates: 10 g, Fiber: 6 g Protein: 6 g

Keto Pull Apart Pizza Bread Recipe

PrepCook Time: 35 minutes, Servings: 16

Ingredients

- 2 1/2 cups Mozzarella Cheese shredded , 3 Eggs beaten
- 1 1/2 cups Almond Flour
- 1 Tbs Baking Powder
- 2 oz Cream Cheese
- 1/2 cup grated Parmesan Cheese
- 1 Tsp Rosemary seasoning
- 1/2 cup shredded mild Cheddar or a cheese or your choice
- 1/2 cup mini pepperoni slices
- Optional: Sliced jalapenos
- Non-stick cooking spray
- Non-stick Bundt Pan I love this Bundt pan found on Amazon

Instructions

- Combine the almond flour with the baking powder until it's fully combined.
- Melt the Mozzarella cheese and cream cheese. You can do this on the stove top or for 1 minute in the microwave.
- Once the cheese has melted, add the flour mixture and eggs and knead it until it forms into a sticky ball. I always use a silicone mat on the countertop to do this step.

- Once the dough has come together and all the ingredients are fully mixed together, sprinkle the top of the dough with a small amount of parmesan cheese. This will help the dough not be so sticky when you start to handle it. I flip the dough over and sprinkle a small amount on the back side of the dough too.
- Form the dough into a ball and cut it in half. Continue cutting the dough until you get about 16 pieces from each side for a total of 32 pieces total (give or take).
- Roll the pieces of dough into equal size balls then roll them in a plate of parmesan cheese that has been topped with a teaspoon of Rosemary seasoning. (This is the secret to forming the pull apart bread because the parmesan cheese coats each dough ball allowing it not to fully combine while it's baking. Plus, it adds amazing flavor to this dough also.)
- Spray the bundt pan with non-stick cooking spray.
- Place the first layer of 16 prepared dough balls into a non-stick bundt pan.
- The add a layer of your favorite shredded cheese, mini pepperoni slices, and jalapenos if desired.
- Add the next layer of 16 prepared dough balls on top of the first layer.
- Top the last layer with the rest of the shredded cheese, mini pepperoni slices, and jalapenos.
- Bake at 350 degrees for 25 minutes or until golden brown. It may take a bit longer if your bundt pan is thicker than the one I used.

Nutrition Info : Calories: 142kcal, Carbohydrates: 3.5g, Protein: 11.1g

Keto Flatbread Recipe

Prep+Cook Time 22 minutes, Servings: 4

Ingredients

- 3/4 cup low moisture mozzarella cheese shredded
- 1 tbsp cream cheese , 1 egg
- 2 tbsp almond flour
- 1/4 cup spinach cooked and drained
- 1/8 tsp garlic powder , salt to taste

Instructions

- Preheat oven to 350 degrees Fahrenheit.
- In a microwave-safe bowl, melt mozzarella cheese and cream cheese in the microwave in 30-second bursts, mixing to combine in between intervals.
- Once the cheese is completely melted and combined, mix in egg, almond flour, and spinach.
- Flatten the mixture out on top of a baking sheet lined with parchment paper. Sprinkle garlic powder and salt on top.

- Bake for 15 minutes, then flip the flatbread to bake for an additional 5 minutes to crisp the other side.

Nutrition Info : Calories 75 Calories from Fat 45 , Total Fat 5g 8% , Saturated Fat 2g 10% , Cholesterol 37mg 12% , Sodium 111mg 5% , Potassium 30mg 1% , Total Carbohydrates 1g 0% , Protein 5g

Zucchini Coconut Bread

Prep+Cook Time 60 minutes, Servings: 6

Ingredients

- 3/4 cup coconut flour
- 1/2 cup zucchini (grated and drained)
- 1/4 cup Pecan (chopped)
- 3/4 tbsp baking powder
- 1 tsp vanilla extract
- 1 scoop unflavored protein powder (around 28 - 30g)
- 6 large eggs
- 1/2 cup butter salted
- 1/2 cup So Nourished Erythritol (or less, up to your liking)
- 1/2 teaspoon salt

Instructions

- Preheat your oven to 350°F.
- Rinse the zucchini well with water and use a hand grater to shred it. Salt the grated zucchini in a bowl. Move to a

o Start making the dry mixture in a bowl. Fold the coconut flour, baking powder, and protein powder with the sweetener. Mix until blended entirely.

o Beat the eggs in a mixer together with vanilla extract and melted butter. Transfer the grated zucchini in and carefully add the dry mixture too. Whisk together until incorporated. Drop the chopped pecan.

o Coat a loaf pan with melted butter. Evenly spread the bread batter into the pan. Place in the oven for 40-45 minutes or until the bread is browned and cooked. Once the surface turns golden, take out from the oven and let sit for 10 minutes before removing from the pan.

o Slice and enjoy!

Nutrition Info: Calories: 160, Fat: 14.3g, Net carbs: 0.9g (total carbs: 1.7g, dietary fiber: 0.8g), Protein: 6.9g

Indian Fry Bread (Low Carb)

Prep+Cook Time 20 mins, Servings: 4 Fry Breads

Ingredients

- 1 ½ Cups Shredded Mozzarella Cheese
- 2 Tablespoons Cream Cheese
- 1 Egg
- 1 Teaspoon Baking Powder
- 1 Cup Almond Flour or you can use Trim Healthy Mama Baking Blend
- 1 ½ Cups Refined Coconut Oil for frying

Instructions

- o Heat coconut oil in a frying pan over medium-low heat.

Make the Dough:

- o In a large microwaveable bowl, melt mozzarella cheese and cream cheese.
- o Stir will, then add egg and baking powder and stir again.
- o Add almond flour, 1/4 cup at a time, stirring well after each addition. (You should have an even,

homogenous dough. You may have to knead it with your hands a bit.)
- o Turn dough onto parchment paper and divide into four balls.
- o Flatten each ball between parchment paper and roll into a 6-8 inch circle with a rolling pin.

Fry the Dough:

- o When the oil has heated, fry dough (one at a time) for about 20 seconds, then flip and fry 20 seconds on the other side. The bread should be a light golden brown color.
- o Remove from oil and drain on paper towels.
- o Serve with all your favorite taco toppings for an Indian Fry Bread Taco!

Nutrition Info : Calories: 589kcal, Carbohydrates: 7g, Protein: 18g, Fat: 55g, Fiber: 3g

Low Carb and Keto Fluffy Waffles Recipe

Prep+Cook Time: 10 minutes, Servings: 4 full waffles

Ingredients

- 4 oz Cream Cheese
- 4 eggs
- 1 tablespoon melted butter
- 1 teaspoon vanilla extract
- 1 tablespoon powdered stevia
- 4 tablespoons coconut flour
- 1 1/2 teaspoons baking powder

Instructions

- Add all the ingredients to a blender and blend it on high for about 1 minute until all the ingredients come out nice and smooth. If you don't have a blender, you can mix it in a small bowl on medium speed for a minute or two. You will want to make sure you cream together all of the cream cheese so you don't have any lumps.
- Optional: Add cinnamon for extra flavor.
- Preheat the waffles iron.
- Spray the waffle iron with non-stick cooking spray.

- Pour about 1/8 to a 1/4 cup batter for each waffle. Note: the batter only spreads a bit more than the amount you put on the waffle iron. It's not like the regular carb filled waffle recipe where you put a small amount on the iron and it's dripping over the edges after a few minutes.
- These are very filling so don't be surprised if you only end up eating 2 out of the 4 waffle squares.
- Optional: Top with butter and sugar-free syrup.

Nutrition Info : Calories: 231kcal, Carbohydrates: 7.7g, Protein: 9.6g, Fat: 18.2g

Low Carb Keto Bagels Recipe (Fathead Dough)

Prep+Cook Time: 22 minutes, Servings: 6

Ingredients

- 1 1/2 cup part-skim shredded mozzarella cheese (about 6 ounces)
- 2 ounces full-fat cream cheese, cut into pieces
- 1 large egg
- 1 1/4 cup almond flour (nut-free options in post) (see conversion chart in site menu)
- 1 tbsp baking powder
- 1 tbsp oat fiber (or 2 tbsp whey protein powder or 1/4 cup more almond flour)*

Instructions

- Place the mozzarella cheese and cream cheese in a microwave safe bowl and microwave for 1 minute. Stir and microwave for 30 seconds to 1 minute more. Scrape the cheese into a food processor with the egg and process until smooth.

- Add the dry ingredients and process until a dough forms. It is very sticky! Scrape onto a piece of cling film and place into the freezer.
- Preheat oven to 400 F and place rack into the middle of the oven. Line a baking sheet with parchment.
- When oven is ready, remove the bagel dough from the freezer and divide into 6 equal pieces. Lightly oil hands and roll each portion into a snake and seal the ends together forming a ring. Place on the parchment paper and top with your favorite topping, pressing gently to adhere.
- Bake for 12 minutes or until the outside has browned. They will still be soft, so let them cool before removing from the baking sheet. Once cool, store in a bag in the refrigerator. Warm slightly to enjoy or toast.
- Makes 6 average sized bagels. Dividing the dough into 8 portions results in mini bagels and dividing into 4 results in gourmet sized bagels. (Don't have a food processor? Read the post for other methods.)
- Keep bagels in the refrigerator in an airtight container. They keep for 7-10 days and also freeze well.

Nutrition Info : Calories 245 Calories from Fat 189 , Total Fat 21g 32% , Sodium 316mg 13% , Total Carbohydrates 6g 2% , Dietary Fiber 3g 12% , Protein 12g

Made in the
USA
Monee, IL